Tofu Recipes

The Ultimate Tofu Cookbook for the Vegetarian

(Everything You Need to Know About Cooking and Eating Tofu Includes Delicious Homemade Recipes)

Daniel Dennis

Published By **Oliver Leish**

Daniel Dennis

Tofu Recipes: The Ultimate Tofu Cookbook for the Vegetarian (Everything You Need to Know About Cooking and Eating Tofu Includes Delicious Homemade Recipes)

ISBN 978-1-998901-80-7

Legal & Disclaimer

Table of Contents

1. BROILED TOFU WITH MISO

Serves four

What you'll want:

1 (14-to sixteen-ounces) block business enterprise tofu, tired

1/three cup purple (darkish) miso (preferably Japanese)

2 tablespoons sugar

2 tablespoons sake, dry Sherry, or dry white wine

1 teaspoon sesame seeds, toasted

Equipment: 12 -pronged wooden alternatives or 24 (2 1/2 of-to 31/2-inch) straight away wood picks

What to do:

Pat tofu dry with paper towels, then wrap in easy paper towels and installation a microwave-secure dish (see chefs' test, underneath). Microwave at immoderate power 30 seconds. Pour off any liquid and wrap tofu in glowing paper towels. Microwave 1 or 2 greater times for 30 seconds every time, pouring off any liquid, until tofu feels more impregnable.

Preheat broiler.

Stir collectively miso, sugar, and sake in a small saucepan. (If miso combination may be very thick, stir in 1 tablespoon water.) Cook over medium-excessive warm temperature, stirring, until bubbling, sleek, and the consistency of ketchup, 1 to three minutes.

Cut tofu in half of of horizontally and installation, reduce sides up, on a slicing board. Cut every half into 6 squares (portions might not be perfectly square).

Arrange tofu on a foil-coated broiler pan, reduce facets up, and broil about 2 inches from heat till a crust just paperwork, 1 to 2 mins. Remove from oven and spread crusted facet of every rectangular with about three/4 teaspoon miso aggregate. Broil until tops are surely bubbling and beginning to shade, 1 to two minutes. Transfer to a plate. Skewer every rectangular with 1 -pronged select out or 2 parallel right now selections. Sprinkle with seeds.

2. SPICY KIMCHI TOFU STEW

Serves 6

What you'll want:

Kosher salt

1 16-ounce bundle silken tofu, lessen into 1" quantities

1 tablespoon vegetable oil

four cups lightly squeezed cabbage kimchi, chopped, plus 1 cup liquid

2 tablespoons gochujang (Korean warm pepper paste)

eight scallions, reduce into 1" portions

2 tablespoons reduced-sodium soy sauce

1 tablespoon toasted sesame oil

Freshly floor black pepper

6 large egg yolks

2 tablespoons toasted sesame seeds

What to do:

Bring a massive pot of salted water to a boil. Reduce warm temperature, cautiously upload tofu, and simmer gently till slightly puffed and firmed up, approximately 4 mins. Using a slotted spoon, switch tofu to a medium bowl.

Heat vegetable oil in a huge heavy pot over medium-excessive warmth. Add kimchi and gochujang and put together dinner, stirring often, till beginning to brown, 5–eight mins. Add kimchi liquid and 8 cups water. Bring to a boil, reduce warmth, and simmer until kimchi is softened and translucent, 35–40 mins.

Add scallions, soy sauce, and tofu; simmer lightly until tofu has absorbed flavors, 20–25 minutes (tofu will fall apart a little). Add sesame oil; season with salt and pepper. Ladle stew into bowls; top each with an egg yolk and sesame seeds.

3. BLACK PEPPER TOFU

Serves 4

What you'll need:

1 3/four lbs enterprise tofu

Vegetable oil for frying

Cornstarch to dirt the tofu

11 tbsp butter

12 small shallots (12 ounces. In desired), thinly sliced

eight easy red chiles (quite slight ones), thinly sliced

12 garlic cloves, beaten

three tbsp chopped smooth ginger

3 tbsp sweet soy sauce (kecap manis)

3 tbsp mild soy sauce

4 tsp dark soy sauce

2 tbsp sugar

five tbsp coarsely overwhelmed black peppercorns (use a mortar and pestle or a spice grinder)

16 small and thin green onions, reduce into 1 1/4-inch segments

What to do:

Start with the tofu. Pour sufficient oil proper right into a massive frying pan or wok to come back again again 1/four inch up the edges and heat. Cut the tofu into huge cubes, approximately 1 x 1 inch. Toss them in some cornstarch and shake off the more, then upload to the current oil. (You'll want to fry the tofu portions in some batches simply so they do no longer stew in the pan.) Fry, turning them round as you pass, until they are golden within the route of and function a skinny crust. As they are cooked, transfer them onto paper towels.

Remove the oil and any sediment from the pan, then positioned the butter inner and melt it. Add the shallots, chiles, garlic and ginger. Sauté on low to medium heat for about 15 mins, stirring now and again, until the factors have have end up vivid and are genuinely mild. Next, add the soy sauces and sugar and stir, then add the beaten black pepper.

Add the tofu to warm temperature it up inside the sauce for approximately a minute. Finally, stir inside the green onions. Serve heat, with steamed rice.

4. PANANG TOFU CURRY

Serves four

What you'll want:

1 1/2 tablespoons olive oil

half of cup finely chopped shallots

2 tablespoons finely grated peeled ginger

4 garlic cloves, finely chopped

1/four cup organic peanut butter

2 teaspoons turmeric

1 teaspoon floor cumin

1 teaspoon warm chili paste (together with sambal oelek)

1 cup water

1 thirteen half of of-to fourteen-ounce can natural light coconut milk

three kaffir lime leaves or 3 tablespoons sparkling lime juice and 1 half of teaspoons finely grated lime peel

1 tablespoon (firmly packed) golden brown sugar

2 14-ounce programs herbal agency tofu, worn-out, reduce into 1-inch cubes 1 1/2 of cups 1/four- to one/3-inch-thick slices peeled carrots (about 3 medium)

1 half of of cups 1/four- to 1/3-inch-thick slices peeled carrots (about three medium)

1 massive crimson bell pepper, reduce into 3/4-inch portions

What to do:

Heat oil in heavy huge skillet over medium-immoderate warm temperature. Add shallots, ginger, and garlic; prepare dinner dinner till shallots are soft, about 6 mins. Add peanut butter, turmeric, cumin, and chili paste; stir till aromatic, 1 to two minutes. Whisk in 1 cup water, then coconut milk, lime leaves, and brown sugar; convey to simmer. Season sauce with salt. Add tofu, carrots, and bell pepper; simmer over medium warm temperature till carrots are mild, adjusting warm temperature to medium-low if starting to boil and on occasion stirring lightly, approximately 20 minutes. Season to taste with salt.

5. TOFU STIR FRY

Serves four

What you'll need:

1 package deal deal (14 oz.) more-enterprise tofu

1 tablespoon soy sauce

1 teaspoon garlic powder

2 tablespoons all-cause flour

2 tablespoons sesame oil

1 small crimson bell pepper, seeded, cored and thinly sliced

1 small green bell pepper, seeded, cored and thinly sliced

6 green onions, reduce into 1/four-inch quantities

1 bundle (eight ounce) complete-wheat lo mein noodles

6 tablespoons white miso paste

2 cloves garlic, minced

1 piece ginger (1 inch), minced

1 teaspoon orange zest

1/4 cup orange juice

1 can (15 ounce) toddler corn, tired and rinsed

1 can (8 ounce) water chestnuts, worn-out and rinsed

What to do:

Place tofu in a colander; set a heavy pot on pinnacle 10 to fifteen minutes to press out moisture. Halve; sprinkle soy sauce, garlic powder, then flour over halves. Heat 1 tablespoon oil over medium-excessive warm temperature in a large skillet.

Cook tofu until golden, 2 to three minutes in line with thing. Slicc; set aside. In identical skillet, prepare dinner peppers and onions, covered, till peppers melt, 7 to 8 mins. Cook noodles as directed on package deal. Whisk miso paste, garlic, ginger, zest, juice and closing 1 tablespoon oil in a bowl. Add pepper combination, noodles, corn, water chestnuts; toss. Top with tofu.

6. TOFU-AND-MEAT LOAF

Serves 6

What you'll need:

For the topping:

three tablespoons ketchup

2 tablespoons hoisin sauce

2 teaspoons Dijon mustard

1/2 tablespoon moderate brown sugar

For the loaf:

1 (14-ounce) package deal deal greater-commercial enterprise business enterprise tofu, worn-out

half of of of pound ground beef

1/2 pound floor turkey

three slices bread, torn into small quantities

2 eggs, lightly beaten

half of onion, finely chopped

1 celery stalk, finely chopped

2 tablespoons soy sauce

2 tablespoons hoisin sauce

1 teaspoon minced garlic

1 teaspoon minced ginger (non-obligatory)

1/four teaspoon crimson pepper flakes (non-obligatory)

What to do:

A day earlier, collapse the tofu right right into a plastic problem. Freeze in a unmarried day or for up to 4 hours. Thaw the tofu and pat it dry with a paper towel earlier than the usage of.

Preheat oven to 350°F. In a small bowl, whisk collectively the topping factors.

In a large bowl, break up the tofu together with your palms. Add the very last loaf substances and integrate nicely. Pat the combination proper right into a 9-by means of way of way of-5-inch loaf pan. Bake for 45 mins.

Remove the loaf and brush it with the topping, then go back it to the oven and bake for 15 minutes greater.

Remove and allow the loaf cool for 5 mins earlier than reducing and serving.

7. TOFU RIGATONI CASSEROLE

Serves 8

What you'll need:

1/four cup extra-virgin olive oil, plus more for drizzling

half of onion, finely chopped

three garlic cloves, finely chopped

1 (28-ounce) can crushed tomatoes

1 pinch dried oregano

1 (12- to fourteen-ounce) package deal agency tofu, worn-out

1 huge egg

1 pinch grated nutmeg

Salt and freshly floor black pepper to flavor

1 (10-ounce) bundle frozen spinach, defrosted and tired

1 (1-pound) container rigatoni, cooked al dente and tired

1 pound fresh mozzarella, grated (about four cups)

three ouncesGrated Parmesan (about 3/four cup)

What to do:

Preheat oven to 350°F.

Heat the oil in a saucepan over medium-excessive warmth. Add the onion. Sauté for three mins, then add the garlic and put together dinner until the onion is translucent, approximately 2 mins more.

Add the tomatoes and oregano. Reduce warm temperature and simmer, stirring on occasion, for 15 mins. Meanwhile, in a blender, way the tofu, egg, nutmeg, salt, and pepper until smooth.

Transfer the aggregate to a bowl and fold in the spinach, cooked rigatoni, tomato sauce, 1 cup of the mozzarella, and 1/2 of of cup of the Parmesan.

Drizzle a coating of olive oil proper right right into a thirteen-with the resource of way of-nine-inch baking pan. Add the pasta mixture and sprinkle the very last cheeses over the top. Bake till golden and effervescent, 35 to forty minutes. Let cool for 10 mins in advance than decreasing.

8. CREAMY TOFU SALAD

Serves 4

What you'll need:

1 (14-oz..) bundle deal business enterprise tofu, rinsed and drained

1/2 of cup mayonnaise

1 teaspoon sparkling lemon juice

1 teaspoon turmeric

half of of teaspoon dry mustard

2 celery ribs, finely chopped

1/4 cup chopped clean chives

1/2 of teaspoon salt, or to flavor

1/4 teaspoon black pepper, or to flavor

Accompaniments: sandwich bread; lettuce leaves; sliced tomato

What to do:

Finely mash tofu with a fork in a bowl, then allow drain in a sieve set over some other bowl, about 15 mins (discard liquid).

While tofu drains, whisk together mayonnaise, lemon juice, turmeric, and mustard in bowl, then stir in tofu, celery, chives, salt, and pepper.

9. TOASTED ALMOND TOFU BURGERS

Serves four

What you'll need:

1 12-ounce bundle deal corporation tofu, tired, patted dry, lessen into 1-inch-thick slices

Nonstick vegetable oil spray

half cup grated carrot

half of cup thinly sliced inexperienced onions

2 teaspoons minced peeled ginger

1 garlic clove, minced

half of cup almonds, toasted, finely chopped

1 big egg white, crushed to combination

4 teaspoons soy sauce

1 teaspoon oriental sesame oil

1 teaspoon sesame seeds, toasted

4 sesame seed buns, toasted

4 tomato slices

1 cup alfalfa sprouts

What to do:

Wrap tofu in doubled dish towel. Place on paintings ground. Weigh down with a board topped with meals cans or weights for 1 hour. Squeeze towel-wrapped tofu to extract as a exquisite deal liquid as possible from tofu. Transfer tofu to medium bowl. Using fork, mash into small portions.

Spray medium nonstick skillet with nonstick spray; area over medium warmth. Add carrot, green onions, ginger and garlic; sauté until barely softened, about 3 minutes. Cool. Mix carrot mixture, almonds, egg white, soy sauce, sesame oil and sesame seeds into tofu. Season with salt and pepper. Shape mixture into 4 1/2 of-inch-thick patties. (Can be made 4 hours beforehand. Cover and sit down again.)

If grilling, spray grill rack with nonstick spray, then prepare fish fry (medium warm temperature). If sautéing, spray big nonstick skillet with nonstick spray and heat over medium warmth. Lightly spray patties on each elements with nonstick spray. Place patties on grill or in skillet and prepare dinner till golden brown and heated through, about 3 minutes consistent with element.

Place 1 burger on every bun bottom. Top each with 1 tomato slice, a few sprouts and bun pinnacle and serve.

10. WARM TOFU WITH SPICY GARLIC SAUCE

Serves eight

What you'll want:

1 (14-to 18-oz) package deal smooth tofu (not silken)

1 teaspoon chopped garlic

1/four cup chopped scallion

2 teaspoons sesame seeds, toasted and beaten with aspect of a heavy knife

3 tablespoons soy sauce

1 tablespoon Asian sesame oil

1 teaspoon coarse Korean heat crimson-pepper flakes

half of teaspoon sugar

What to do:

Carefully rinse tofu, then cover with bloodless water in a medium saucepan. Bring to a simmer over medium-excessive warm temperature, then hold heat, blanketed, over very low heat.

Meanwhile, mince and mash garlic to a paste with a pinch of salt. Stir collectively with ultimate factors (except tofu).

Just earlier than serving, cautiously carry tofu from saucepan with a large spatula and drain on paper towels. Gently pat dry, then transfer to a small plate. Spoon a few sauce over tofu and serve warmth. Serve closing sauce on

11. PANFRIED TOFU WITH ASIAN CARAMEL SAUCE

Serves four

What you'll want:

1 (14-ounce) block extra-business business enterprise tofu, rinsed

half pound shallots (four to 5 large)

1 cup vegetable oil

1/three cup sugar

1 garlic clove, finely chopped

half of tablespoon finely chopped peeled glowing ginger

24

3 tablespoons soy sauce

3 tablespoons rice vinegar (not pro)

1 1/three cups plus 2 tablespoons water

2 tablespoons cornstarch

1/3 cup loosely packed smooth basil leaves

1/three cup loosely packed clean mint leaves

Cooked jasmine rice; steamed infant bok choy (non-obligatory); lime wedges

What to do:

Drain tofu and fry shallots:

Halve tofu crosswise, then lessen lengthwise into fourths to form 8 slices. Put tofu slices among numerous layers of paper towels to empty, changing towels as needed, till organized to apply.

Finely chop sufficient shallots to diploma 1/2 cup and reserve. Cut very last shallots crosswise into 1/eight-inch-thick slices and separate into rings. Heat oil in a 10-inch heavy skillet (ideally cast-iron) over fairly high warmth till heat but no longer smoking, then fry sliced shallots in 2 batches, stirring now and again, till golden brown, 1 half of of to a few minutes consistent with batch (watch carefully, as shallots can burn without difficulty). Quickly switch shallots as fried with a slotted spoon to paper towels to drain. Pour off all however 1 tablespoon oil from skillet and reserve skillet.

Make sauce:

Cook sugar in a dry 1- to at the least one half of-quart heavy saucepan over moderate heat, undisturbed, till it melts round edges and starts offevolved to reveal golden, then maintain to cook, stirring, until all of sugar is melted and turns a golden caramel.

Add reserved chopped shallots (use warning; caramel will bubble up and steam vigorously) and prepare dinner dinner, stirring, till shallots reduce returned and are very aromatic, approximately forty five seconds. Add garlic and ginger and prepare dinner dinner, stirring, 30 seconds. Stir in soy sauce, vinegar, and 1 1/three cups water and simmer, stirring, until any hardened caramel is dissolved, approximately 1 minute.

Stir together cornstarch and closing 2 tablespoons water until smooth, then stir into sauce and simmer, stirring now and again, 2 minutes. Remove from warmth and keep warm, included.

Panfry tofu:

Heat oil very last in skillet over high warmth until warmness but not smoking. Meanwhile, blot any extra moisture ultimate on tofu with paper towels, then upload to warmth oil in skillet in 1 layer. Fry tofu, turning over once, until golden and crisp, 7 to ten mins overall. Transfer to easy paper towels to empty briefly.

Reheat sauce, then serve tofu crowned with sauce, basil, mint, and fried shallots.

12. MARINATED TOFU WITH PEANUTS AND CHARRED BEAN SPROUTS

Serves four

What you'll want:

2 14-ounce applications organisation tofu, tired, sliced half of" thick

1 jalapeño, with seeds, thinly sliced

half of of cup reduced-sodium soy sauce

2 tablespoons mild brown sugar

2 teaspoons grated peeled ginger

2 teaspoons vegetable oil

2 cups bean sprouts, divided

Kosher salt

Steamed white rice (for serving)

6 scallions, thinly sliced on a diagonal

half of cup chopped salted, roasted peanuts

1/4 cup sparkling mint leaves

Lime wedges (for serving)

What to do:

Place tofu on a baking sheet blanketed with numerous layers of paper towels; area severa layers of paper towels on top and press gently to squeeze out liquid. Cut tofu into three/four"-massive portions and area in a baking dish.

Whisk jalapeño, soy sauce, brown sugar, and ginger in a small bowl, pour over tofu, and toss to coat. Let take a seat down at least half of of-hour.

Just earlier than serving, warm temperature oil in a medium skillet over medium-excessive warmth. Add 1 cup bean sprouts and cook dinner, undisturbed, until charred, approximately three minutes; season with salt.

Spoon tofu over rice and pinnacle with charred and uncooked bean sprouts, scallions, peanuts, and mint. Serve with lime wedges.

13. PANFRIED TOFU WITH ROMANO-BEAN AND HERB SALAD

Serves 6

What you'll want:

2 (14-ounces.) applications clean tofu (no longer silken)

6 big eggs (four hard-boiled and 2 uncooked)

2 tablespoons smooth lemon juice

2 tablespoons water

1 tablespoon Dijon mustard

1/2 of cup plus 2 tablespoon vegetable oil, divided

1 medium shallot, minced (2 tablespoons)

1/three cup chopped flat-leaf parsley

2 tablespoons tired capers, chopped

1 half of kilos Romano beans or green beans, trimmed

five ounces wild or toddler arugula (6 packed cups)

1/3 cup tarragon leaves

What to do:

Cut each tofu block lengthwise into three equal portions. Drain on paper towels.

Peel hard-boiled eggs and halve lengthwise. Remove difficult-boiled yolks and location in a meals processor. Thinly slice whites crosswise and reserve.

Add lemon juice, water, mustard, and 1/4 teaspoon every of salt and pepper to yolks in meals processor. With motor going for walks, upload 1/2 of cup oil in a sluggish circulate, processing till emulsified and clean and scraping down elements as preferred. Transfer to a bowl and stir in shallot, parsley, and capers. Reserve 1/four cup dressing for serving.

Cook beans, uncovered, in well-salted boiling water tlll crisp-tender, 4 to five minutes. Transfer to an ice tub to prevent cooking, then drain well. Transfer to a bowl and toss with dressing (excluding 1/4 reserved dressing for serving). Gently toss with arugula, tarragon, and egg whites. Season with salt and pepper.

Heat ultimate 2 tablespoons oil in a 12-inch nonstick skillet over medium warm temperature. Meanwhile, lightly beat closing 2 eggs in a medium bowl. Pat tofu dry and season every additives with half of of teaspoon salt (normal). Coat tofu with egg, letting greater drip off, then fry, turning as soon as, until golden and heated via, 8 to ten mins. Drain in quick on paper towels, then serve with salad and reserved dressing.

14. MA–PO TOFU (SPICY BEAN CURD WITH BEEF)

Serves 4

What you'll need:

1 teaspoon Sichuan peppercorns

1 half of pounds mild (no longer silken) tofu, lessen into 1-inch cubes

2 tablespoons Chinese heat bean paste (additionally called chili bean sauce)*

1 tablespoon Chinese black-bean paste or sauce*

four tablespoons oyster sauce

2 tablespoons Asian chili powder*

1 tablespoon cornstarch

1/four cup peanut oil

4 ozground beef

1 (1/four-inch) piece sparkling ginger, minced (about 1 teaspoon)

2 cloves garlic, minced

1 scallion (white and inexperienced elements), thinly sliced on diagonal

1/four cup Shaohsing rice wine

1 medium leek (white and slight green additives nice), washed, halved

lengthwise, and cut into half-inch slices (approximately half of cup)

1/2 cup hen inventory or low-sodium fowl broth

1 tablespoon mild soy sauce

1 tablespoon dark soy sauce

2 tablespoons sparkling cilantro, chopped (non-obligatory)

What to do:

In dry heavy skillet over moderate warmth, toast peppercorns, stirring, till fragrant, three to 5 minutes. Transfer to bowl and allow cool, then grind in spice grinder to pleasant powder. Set aside.

In big pot over fairly immoderate warmth, carry four cups water to boil. Add tofu, put off from warm temperature, and allow steep, uncovered, 5 mins. Using slotted spoon, transfer tofu to medium bowl and set apart.

In small bowl, whisk collectively hot bean paste, black-bean paste, 2 tablespoons oyster sauce, and chili powder. Set aside.

In small bowl, whisk together cornstarch and three tablespoons water. Set aside.

In wok or heavy big sauté pan over slight warmness, warmth oil till warmness but now not smoking. Add beef, ginger, garlic, and scallions and stir-fry until meat is browned, approximately 1 minute. Add rice wine and put together dinner, stirring occasionally, till maximum of moisture evaporates, 1 to two mins. Add heat bean paste aggregate and prepare dinner, stirring on occasion, till aggregate is blanketed and oil in pan turns red, about 1 minute.

Add tofu, leeks, inventory, mild and dark soy sauces, and very last 2 tablespoons oyster sauce and convey to boil. Whisk cornstarch combination to recombine, then add to pan and put together dinner, stirring every now and then, till juices thicken barely, about 1 minute.

Transfer to serving dish. Sprinkle with Sichuan peppercorn powder and cilantro, if the usage of. Serve without delay.

15. SPICY THAI TOFU WITH RED BELL PEPPERS AND PEANUTS

Serves four

What you'll need:

1/three cup olive oil

2 huge pink bell peppers, seeded, thinly sliced

3 tablespoons minced peeled sparkling ginger

3 huge garlic cloves, finely chopped

1 14-to sixteen-ounce package deal extra-corporation tofu, worn-out well, reduce into 1-inch cubes

three inexperienced onions, thinly sliced on diagonal

three tablespoons soy sauce

2 tablespoons easy lime juice

half to three/four teaspoon dried beaten purple pepper

1 6-ounce bag little one spinach leaves

1/3 cup chopped sparkling basil

1/3 cup lightly salted roasted peanuts

What to do:

Heat oil in wok over high warmth. Add bell peppers, ginger, and garlic; sauté until peppers just begin to melt, about 2 mins. Add tofu and inexperienced onions; toss 2 mins. Add next three factors. Toss to mixture, about 1 minute. Add spinach in 3 additions, tossing until starting to wilt, approximately 1 minute for every addition. Mix in basil. Season with salt and pepper. Sprinkle peanuts over.

16. FIVE-SPICE TOFU STIR-FRY WITH CARROTS AND CELERY

Serves four

What you'll want:

2 tablespoons peanut oil or vegetable oil, divided

8 oz... Savory baked five-spice tofu cakes (approximately 2 squares), cut into matchstick-length strips

2 cups matchstick-length strips carrots (approximately 3 medium)

2 cups matchstick-period strips celery (approximately 3 prolonged stalks)

1/three cup finely chopped rinsed canned Szechuan preserved vegetable (about 1 1/4 oz..)

1 tablespoon Shaoxing wine (Chinese rice wine) or dry Sherry

half of teaspoon salt

half of teaspoon sugar

1/4 teaspoon floor white pepper

2 teaspoons Asian sesame oil

What to do:

Heat 14-inch-diameter flat-bottomed wok or heavy 12-inch-diameter skillet over immoderate warm temperature until drop of water delivered to wok evaporates on contact. Add 1 tablespoon peanut oil and swirl, then upload tofu and stir-fry until tofu honestly starts offevolved to brown, approximately 1 minute.

Transfer tofu to plate. Add final 1 tablespoon peanut oil to identical wok (do no longer easy). Add carrots, celery, and Szechuan preserved vegetable and stir-fry till carrots are crisp-easy, about three minutes. Return tofu to wok; add rice wine, salt, sugar, and white pepper. Stir-fry to aggregate, approximately 1 minute. Remove pan from warm temperature; stir in sesame oil and serve.

17. SPICY LIME AND HERBED TOFU IN LETTUCE CUPS

Serves 6

What you'll need:

Dressing:

1/4 cup thinly sliced peeled glowing ginger

1/4 cup thinly sliced sparkling lemongrass, cut from bottom 4 inches of 4 stalks with difficult leaves removed

1/four cup fresh lime juice

2 tablespoons fish sauce (which consist of nam pla or nuoc nam)

2 tablespoons water

three tablespoons candy chili sauce*

Tofu:

half of cup diced seeded peeled cucumber

1/4 cup chopped inexperienced onions

1/four cup diced seeded plum tomato

2 tablespoons chopped seeded jalapeño chile

1 tablespoon finely chopped sparkling cilantro

1 tablespoon finely chopped clean mint

1 tablespoon finely chopped easy basil (preferably Vietnamese or Thai)

1 14- to 16-ounce bundle deal company tofu, worn-out, reduce into 1/2 of-inch cubes, patted dry

6 large or 12 medium butter lettuce leaves

What to do:

For dressing:

Puree first 5 elements in blender. Let mixture stand as a minimum 15 minutes and up to at the least one hour. Strain aggregate into small bowl, urgent on solids to release any liquid; discard solids. Stir in sweet chili sauce. (Can be made 1 day in advance. Cover and refrigerate.)

For tofu:

Combine first 7 materials in massive bowl. Add tofu and dressing to bowl; toss to coat.

Arrange 1 or 2 lettuce leaves on each of 6 plates. Divide tofu aggregate among lettuce leaves and serve.

18. THAI TOFU WITH ZUCCHINI, RED BELL PEPPER, AND LIME

Serves 4

What you'll want:

2 tablespoons peanut oil, divided

1 12-ounce package deal greater-organisation tofu, tired, patted dry, reduce into half of-inch cubes

1 pound yellow and/or inexperienced zucchini, reduce into half of-inch cubes

1 big pink bell pepper, diced

1 tablespoon minced peeled clean ginger

1 1/three cups canned unsweetened coconut milk

three tablespoons (or extra) glowing lime juice

1 half of tablespoons soy sauce

three/four teaspoon Thai crimson curry paste

half of of cup sliced clean basil, divided

What to do:

Heat 1 tablespoon oil in big nonstick skillet over medium-immoderate warm temperature. Add tofu; sauté till golden, about 4 minutes. Transfer tofu to bowl. Add remaining 1 tablespoon oil, then zucchini and bell pepper to skillet; sauté until beginning to melt, about 4 mins. Return tofu to skillet. Add ginger; stir 30 seconds.

Add coconut milk, three tablespoons lime juice, soy sauce, and curry paste; stir to dissolve curry paste. Simmer until sauce thickens, about 6 minutes. Season with salt and extra lime juice, if preferred. Stir in half of of of of basil. Sprinkle with last basil; serve.

19. COCONUT CURRIED TOFU WITH GREEN JASMINE RICE

Serves four

What you'll need:

1/4 cup unsweetened shredded coconut

1 3/4 cups water

1 teaspoon salt

1 cup jasmine or basmati rice

1 cup (packed) coarsely chopped sparkling cilantro

3/four cup unsweetened mild coconut milk

four teaspoons minced easy ginger

1 tablespoon easy lime juice

2 massive garlic cloves, minced

2 tablespoons vegetable oil

sixteen ouncesextra-organization tofu, tired, patted dry, lessen into 1/2 of-inch cubes

1/2 cup thinly sliced inexperienced onions

2 teaspoons curry powder

1 teaspoon ground cumin

1/8 teaspoon dried crushed red pepper

1 cup complete small cherry tomatoes

2 tablespoons chopped peanuts

What to do:

Stir shredded coconut in small nonstick skillet over medium warm temperature until slight golden, about five minutes. Transfer to bowl.

Bring 1 3/4 cups water and salt to boil in heavy medium saucepan. Stir in rice; carry to boil. Reduce warm temperature to low, cowl, and simmer till water is absorbed and rice is tender, approximately 18 minutes.

Meanwhile, puree cilantro, half cup coconut milk, 1 teaspoon ginger, lime juice, and 1/2 of garlic in blender. Mix puree and coconut into rice. Set apart.

Heat oil in big nonstick skillet over immoderate warmness. Add tofu; stir-fry until golden, about 6 mins. Add onions, curry, cumin, crimson pepper, final ginger, and final garlic. Stir-fry 1 minute. Stir in tomatoes and very last coconut milk. Season with salt and pepper.

Divide rice amongst four plates. Top with tofu combination. Sprinkle with peanuts.

20. PANFRIED TOFU WITH CHINESE BLACK BEAN SAUCE

Serves four

What you'll want:

1-pound block of extra-business enterprise tofu

four garlic cloves

1-inch bite of easy ginger

2 tablespoons Chinese fermented black beans

11/2 cups water

4 tablespoons soy sauce

three tablespoons Sherry (dry or candy)

1 tablespoon maple syrup

2 teaspoons cider vinegar

1 half of tablespoons cornstarch

Vegetable oil

What to do:

Rinse the tofu, then reduce crosswise into 6 slices. Put slices among numerous layers of paper towels and allow drain at the same time as making the sauce. (You'll probably have to replace the paper towels as a minimum as quickly as.)

Prep the seasonings for the sauce: Peel the garlic cloves and the ginger, then vicinity the ginger. Turn in your food processor and drop the garlic and ginger via the feed tube; they'll be minced in no time. Stop the device and the black beans in a small sieve till the water runs smooth. Add them to the food processor and pulse until coarsely chopped.

For the liquid part of the sauce, stir collectively the water, soy sauce, Sherry, maple syrup, vinegar, and the cornstarch till the cornstarch is frivolously suspended. Now you're equipped to prepare dinner the sauce!

Generously film the bottom of a heavy 2-quart saucepan with the vegetable oil and heat over reasonably immoderate warmth until heat however not smoking. Stir-fry the seasonings till fragrant, a good deal much less than a minute. Stir the cornstarch mixture and upload it to the pan. Whisk the sauce every so often on the identical time as bringing it to a boil and simmer 1 minute. Then set the sauce apart whilst you fry the tofu.

Generously film the lowest of a 12-inch nonstick skillet with vegetable oil and warmth over high warm temperature until warm but no longer smoking. Blot up any more moisture at the tofu with a paper towel in advance than laying inside the skillet. Fry the slices on all sides (forgo the quick ends), turning them pleasant at the same time as the undersides are golden and crisp, 5 to eight mins regularly occurring. (You may also want to decrease the warm temperature because the frying progresses.) Give the tofu one remaining flip on a paper towel to sop up any stray oil and reheat the sauce.

Serve with rice and broccoli, pouring sauce over all.

21. MISO SOUP WITH VEGETABLES AND TOFU

Serves 4

What you'll want:

2 1/2 of tablespoons purple miso (or greater to flavor)

1 huge clove garlic, chopped

1 teaspoon finely grated ginger

1 half of tablespoons rice wine vinegar, divided

half of of pound enterprise tofu, reduce into cubes

1/4 pound snow peas, trimmed

four massive radishes, thinly sliced

4 scallions, thinly sliced

1 cup pea shoots, sunflower sprouts or radish sprouts

2 teaspoons toasted sesame oil

What to do:

Blend miso with garlic, ginger, 1 cup cool water and 1 tablespoon vinegar in a food processor till clean. Transfer miso broth to a bowl; stir in 2 cups cool water. Divide broth, tofu, snow peas, radishes and scallions among 4 bowls. Toss pea shoots with last 1/2 tablespoon vinegar and oil; garnish every bowl in advance than serving.

22. SALT AND PEPPER TOFU

Serves 2

What you'll want:

1/2 of cup lump crabmeat

1 celery stalk, diced

half of tablespoon chervil, chopped

1 teaspoon finely grated lemon zest

2 avocados

1 cup vegetable inventory

2 tablespoons crème fraîche

1 tablespoon glowing lime juice

three/four teaspoons kosher salt

What to do:

Cut the tofu into 1 half of of with the aid
of 3/four-inch portions and area on a cloth
to dry. Put enough oil in a wok to deep-fry
the tofu and warmth to 350°F, or until a
cube of bread dropped in the oil browns in
15 seconds. Deep-fry the tofu for about

five minutes, or until it's miles golden and truely crisp. Once all of the tofu is cooked, get rid of the oil from the wok and reserve for later use.

Place 2 teaspoons of oil returned into the wok and place over excessive warm temperature. Add the scallions, chile, and garlic, stir-fry for 30 seconds, then go back the tofu to the wok. Toss to mix the flavors and season with the salt and pepper seasoning combination.

23. VEGETABLE AND TOFU RED CURRY

Serves 4

What you'll need:

1 cup jasmine rice

1 three/4 cups water

1 medium onion, halved lengthwise, then thinly sliced crosswise

1 tablespoon vegetable oil

1 massive garlic clove, chopped

2 teaspoons bottled Asian red-curry paste along with Thai Kitchen emblem

1 (14-ounces) can unsweetened coconut milk (no longer low-fat)

1 teaspoon salt

1 (1-lb) package deal frozen combined greens such as broccoli, corn, and crimson peppers

1 (14- to sixteen-oz..) block corporation tofu, rinsed, patted dry, and decrease into half-inch cubes

1 tablespoon Asian fish sauce

Accompaniments: sparkling cilantro sprigs; lime wedges

What to do:

Rinse rice in quick in a sieve and drain, shaking sieve to do away with extra water. Bring rice and 1 1/2 of cups water to a boil in a 1 half of of- to 2-quart heavy saucepan over immoderate warmth, then cover pan with a decent-becoming lid and prepare dinner dinner rice over low warmth until water is absorbed and rice is straightforward, approximately 15 mins.

Meanwhile, cook onion in oil in a huge four-quart heavy pot over reasonably excessive warm temperature, stirring every now and then, until dwindled golden, about three minutes. Reduce warm temperature to moderate, then upload garlic and curry paste and cook dinner, stirring, 1 minute. Stir in coconut milk, salt, and final 1/four cup water and bring to a boil. Stir in veggies and go decrease returned to a boil. Cover pot, then lessen warmth and prepare dinner at a brisk simmer, stirring sometimes, 2 minutes. Gently stir in tofu and simmer curry, in part blanketed, until vegetables are clean, 7 to eight mins. Remove pot from warmness and stir in fish sauce and salt to taste. Serve curry with rice.

24. CURRIED VEGETABLE AND TOFU COUSCOUS

Serves four

What you'll need:

1 5.7-ounce box curried couscous blend

1/2 cup currants

3 tablespoons olive oil

1 12-ounce package greater-employer tofu, drained, patted dry, reduce into half of-inch cubes

three cups broccoli florets

1 medium-period onion, chopped

1 medium-length red bell pepper, coarsely chopped

half of cup water

three/4 cup chopped easy cilantro, divided

What to do:

Following bundle deal pointers, prepare curried couscous. Add currants whilst couscous steams.

Heat olive oil in very big heavy skillet over medium warmth. Add tofu in unmarried layer and prepare dinner without stirring until certainly golden, about 4 minutes. Turn tofu over and put together dinner 2 minutes longer. Transfer tofu to couscous. Add broccoli, onion, and bell pepper to skillet; prepare dinner dinner over medium-excessive warmth 2 mins without stirring.

Continue to prepare dinner vegetables till crisp-gentle, stirring continuously, about 4 mins. Add 1/2 of cup water; growth heat to immoderate and produce to boil, stirring to scrape up browned bits. Mix in 1/2 of cup cilantro. Season vegetables to flavor with salt and pepper. Mix couscous, veggies, and cooking liquid in huge serving bowl. Garnish with remaining 1/4 cup cilantro and serve.

25. LEMONGRASS TOFU WITH MUSHROOMS

Serves 2

What you'll want:

Vegetable oil (for frying)

14 ounces employer tofu, tired, reduce into 3/4-inch squares

3 tablespoons vegetable oil

2 tablespoons minced easy lemongrass

2 garlic cloves, minced

1 teaspoon (heaping) chopped seeded jalapeño chili

1 onion, thinly sliced

half red bell pepper, reduce into 3/four-inch portions

four ouncesshiitake mushrooms, stemmed, thickly sliced

2 teaspoons fish sauce (nuoc mam)

1 tablespoon sugar

1 half tablespoons chopped clean cilantro

What to do:

Add sufficient vegetable oil to heavy medium saucepan to reap intensity of two inches. Heat vegetable oil over medium-excessive warmth to 350°F. Deep-fry tofu squares in 2 batches until golden, about 2 mins. Using slotted spoon, switch tofu to paper towels to drain. Sprinkle with salt and pepper.

Heat three tablespoons vegetable oil in heavy large skillet over medium warmth. Add minced lemongrass, minced garlic, and chopped jalapeño; sauté until fragrant, about 1 minute. Add sliced onion, crimson bell pepper, and sliced shiitake mushrooms; sauté until vegetables are crisp-mild, approximately 3 mins. Add fish sauce and sugar; sauté 1 minute. Add fried tofu squares and sauté till heated through, approximately 1 minute. Transfer to bowl. Sprinkle with chopped sparkling cilantro and serve.

26. SOUTHWESTERN TOFU WRAPS

Serves four

What you'll want:

4 tablespoons easy lime juice

1 tablespoon vegetable oil

eight oz. Firm tofu, tired, patted dry, crumbled

half of of cup chopped crimson onion

1/three cup chopped sparkling cilantro

1 garlic clove, minced

4 7- to eight-inch-diameter flour tortillas

2 cups thinly sliced lettuce leaves

1 cup rather spiced tomato salsa

What to do:

Whisk three tablespoons lime juice and oil in medium bowl. Add tofu, onion, cilantro and garlic and toss to mixture. Season to taste with salt and pepper. Let marinate 20 minutes.

Preheat oven to 350°F. Wrap tortillas in foil. Place in oven until heated through, about 10 mins. Meanwhile, toss lettuce with 1 tablespoon lime juice in small bowl.

Place 1 tortilla on every of 4 plates. Place layer of lettuce down middle of each tortilla. Top with tofu aggregate, dividing in addition. Spoon 1 half of tablespoons salsa over every. Roll up tortillas. Serve, passing remaining salsa one after the opposite.

27. RED LENTIL AND TOFU CURRY

Serves 2

What you'll need:

1 small onion

1 garlic clove

a 1/2 of-inch piece easy gingerroot

half cup red lentils

2 tablespoons vegetable oil

three half of cups water

half of of pound enterprise tofu

half of teaspoon cumin seeds

half teaspoon garam masala or curry powder

half of teaspoon salt

a generous pinch cayenne

3 tablespoons chopped glowing cilantro sprigs

Accompaniment: cooked rice

What to do:

Thinly slice onion and mince garlic. Peel gingerroot and mince. In a sieve rinse lentils and drain. In a 2-quart heavy saucepan prepare dinner dinner onion and garlic in 1 tablespoon oil over mild warmth, stirring, until golden. Add gingerroot and cook dinner, stirring, 1 minute. Add lentils and water and lightly boil, exposed, until lentils disintegrate, approximately 20 minutes.

While lentils are boiling, rinse tofu and trim ends. Cut tofu into 1/2-inch cubes and gently press amongst paper towels to eliminate greater moisture.

In a small heavy skillet heat last tablespoon oil over moderate warmth till warm but not smoking and put together dinner cumin seeds, stirring, until a colour darker, about 1 minute. Add garam masala, salt, and cayenne and prepare dinner, stirring, till aromatic, 15 to 30 seconds. Stir warm spice oil into lentils and gently stir in tofu cubes. Let curry stand, included, five minutes to allow flavors to amplify. Stir in cilantro and salt to flavor.

Serve curry over rice.

28. SPICY TOFU BURRITOS

Serves four

What you'll need:

4 7- to 8-inch-diameter fats-loose flour tortillas

1 tablespoon olive oil

half cup chopped onion

1 half of teaspoons ground cumin

half of teaspoon turmeric

12 ounces. Firm tofu, crumbled (approximately 2 cups)

1 cup chopped red bell pepper

1 half of tablespoons minced seeded jalapeño chili

1 garlic clove, minced

1/2 of of cup grated mozzarella cheese (approximately 2 oz..)

1 cup (packed) thinly sliced romaine lettuce

6 tablespoons chopped easy cilantro

four lime wedges

What to do:

Preheat oven to 350°F. Wrap tortillas in foil. Place in oven until heated through, about 15 mins.

Meanwhile, warmth oil in big nonstick skillet over medium-excessive warmth. Add onion and sauté until golden, approximately five minutes. Add cumin and turmeric; stir 30 seconds. Add tofu, bell pepper, jalapeño and garlic and sauté till heated via, about 3 minutes. Add cheese and stir till melted, about 1 minute. Season to flavor with salt and pepper.

Spoon tofu aggregate down middle of each tortilla, dividing tofu further. Top with lettuce and cilantro. Squeeze juice from lime wedges over. Wrap tortilla round filling and serve.

29. STIR-FRIED TOFU WITH MUSHROOMS, SUGAR SNAP PEAS, AND GREEN ONIONS

Serves four

What you'll need:

3 tablespoons soy sauce

1 tablespoon unseasoned rice vinegar

1 tablespoon honey

1 teaspoon oriental sesame oil

1/4 teaspoon dried overwhelmed purple pepper

1 12-ounce package deal greater-agency tofu, tired, cut into three/4-inch cubes, patted dry with paper towels

1/4 cup water

1 teaspoon cornstarch

2 tablespoons vegetable oil, divided

6 oz.. Clean shiitake mushrooms, stemmed, caps quartered

8 ounces. Sugar snap peas, trimmed

4 garlic cloves, minced

1 tablespoon minced peeled smooth ginger

four inexperienced onions, sliced on diagonal

What to do:

Whisk first 5 materials in medium bowl to combination. Add tofu and stir to coat; allow marinate 1/2-hour. Drain, reserving marinade in small bowl. Whisk 1/four cup water and cornstarch into marinade.

Heat 1 tablespoon vegetable oil in large nonstick skillet over medium-excessive warmness. Add tofu and sauté till golden, approximately 2 minutes. Using slotted spoon, switch tofu to plate. Add very last 1 tablespoon vegetable oil to skillet. Add mushrooms and stir-fry till gentle, about 3 mins. Add sugar snap peas; stir-fry 2 minutes. Add garlic and ginger; stir-fry 30 seconds. Return tofu to skillet; drizzle reserved marinade mixture over. Stir-fry till marinade thickens barely, approximately 30 seconds. Season to taste with salt and pepper. Transfer to bowl. Sprinkle with inexperienced onions and serve.

30. GRILLED TOFU AND SAUTEED ASIAN GREENS

Serves 2

What you'll want:

1 (14-ounce) block organization tofu, drained

1/four cup low-sodium soy sauce

1 teaspoon Asian sesame oil

1 half of teaspoons packed darkish brown sugar

1 half of teaspoons finely grated peeled sparkling ginger

1 small garlic clove, minced

1/four teaspoon Tabasco or dried hot pink pepper flakes

1 tablespoon plus 1 teaspoon vegetable oil

2 (5-ounce) luggage Asian vegetables or infant spinach

What to do:

Cut tofu crosswise into 6 slices. Arrange in 1 layer on a triple layer of paper towels and pinnacle with each distinct triple layer of towels. Weight with a shallow baking pan or baking sheet and allow stand 2 minutes. Repeat weighting with dry paper towels 2 more instances.

Stir together soy sauce, sesame oil, brown sugar, ginger, garlic, Tabasco, and 1 tablespoon vegetable oil in a tumbler pie plate. Add tofu slices in 1 layer and marinate, turning over every short whilst, eight mins ordinary.

Heat a lightly oiled nicely-seasoned ridged grill pan over pretty excessive warmth until heat but not smoking. Lift tofu from marinade with a slotted spatula (reserve marinade) and grill, turning over as soon as cautiously with spatula, until grill marks appear and tofu is heated through, four to 6 minutes today's.

While tofu grills, warmth final teaspoon vegetable oil in a 12-inch skillet over pretty high warmth till hot however now not smoking, then sauté veggies, tossing with tongs, till beginning to wilt. Add reserved marinade and sauté, tossing, till vegetables are surely wilted, about 1 minute. Lift veggies from skillet with tongs, letting extra marinade drip off, and divide amongst 2 plates.

Serve vegetables with tofu slices.

31. SPICY SICHUAN TOFU

Serves 4

What you'll need:

half teaspoon Sichuan peppercorns, toasted and cooled

1 (14- to 17-ounce) package deal deal tofu (no longer silken), rinsed

three tablespoons peanut or vegetable oil

five ounce ground red meat butt (now not lean; 2/three cup)

2 half of tablespoons toban jiang (warm bean sauce)

1 tablespoon fermented black beans, rinsed, worn-out, and chopped

2 teaspoon Asian chile powder

1 cup hen inventory or reduced-sodium chook broth

2 teaspoon soy sauce

1 teaspoon sugar

1 tablespoons cornstarch

4 teaspoons water

four scallions, chopped (half cup)

What to do:

Grind peppercorns in grinder and set aside.

Cut tofu into 3/4-inch cubes and pat dry.

Heat wok over immoderate warmth until it starts offevolved to smoke, then pour oil down facet and swirl to coat backside and side. Stir-fry pork till not pink. Add bean sauce, black beans, and chile powder and stir-fry 1 minute. Stir in stock, soy sauce, sugar, tofu, and a pinch of salt. Simmer, gently stirring sometimes, 5 minutes.

Meanwhile, stir collectively cornstarch and water till easy.

Stir cornstarch mixture into stir-fry and simmer, gently stirring every so often, 1 minute. Stir in scallions and simmer 1 minute. Serve sprinkled with Sichuan pepper.

Serve with steamed rice

32. Sesame Tofu

Serves 4

What you'll want:

14 ozextra business enterprise tofu

1/four cup cornstarch, for dusting

canola oil (for frying)

1/2 cup sesame seeds, gently toasted

1 bunch scallion, trimmed and decrease into 1-inch quantities

Sauce:

1/3 cup honey

3 tablespoons tamari soy sauce

three tablespoons finely minced gingerroot

2 tablespoons sesame oil

2 tablespoons rice wine vinegar

2 finely minced garlic cloves

1 -2 teaspoon purple chili pepper flakes

What to do:

Wrap tofu with paper towels and area on a reducing board.

Put a heavy plate on pinnacle to press out liquid for about 20 minutes.

Stir sauce additives collectively in a saucepan.

Simmer sauce whilst you put together dinner the tofu.

Dry drained tofu with paper towels and dice.

Dust very gently with cornstarch.

Heat 1" oil in deep frying pan.

Fry tofu in 350 diploma F oil till golden brown.

Place fried tofu in a big bowl and toss with 2/three cup sauce, sprinkle liberally with sesame seeds and scallions.

Toss lightly.

Serve final sauce for dipping or drizzled over veggies.

33. Marinated Baked Tofu

Serves 2

What you'll want:

1 (16 ounce) package deal deal enterprise agency tofu or 1 (sixteen ounce) package deal more company tofu, in water

three -4 tablespoons soy sauce

1 -2 minced garlic clove, to taste

1 tablespoon sparkling grated ginger, to taste

1 tablespoon sesame oil

1 tablespoon rice vinegar

1 -2 teaspoon honey (non-obligatory) or 1 -2 teaspoon sugar (non-compulsory)

1 tablespoon olive oil

What to do:

Drain tofu and decrease into 1" cubes.

Mix all other materials together besides olive oil.

Pour marinade over tofu and cowl.

Refrigerate in a unmarried day or longer.

Lightly grease baking pan or sheet with olive oil.

Arrange tofu in unmarried layer on sheet, ensuring now not to forget about the garlic and ginger from the marinade dish.

Bake at 350 tiers for fifty-60 minutes, flipping tofu as a minimum as soon as in a few unspecified time inside the destiny of the method, until brown and slightly crispy.

34. Soy Glazed Tofu and Asparagus

Serves 2

What you'll need:

2 tablespoons sesame oil

1/2 teaspoon cayenne chili pepper flakes

8 stalks asparagus, woody ends snapped off

2/3 cup more organization tofu, reduce into 1/2 of of inch cubes

1 cup sliced button mushroom

1 clove garlic, minced

2 teaspoons granulated sugar

2 tablespoons soy sauce

What to do:

Heat sesame oil and red pepper flakes in nonstick skillet or wok.

Cut asparagus spears into 1 1/2 of inch quantities.

Add asparagus and tofu to heated sesame oil and stir-fry for five minutes.

Add mushrooms and cook dinner dinner for 3 minutes.

Add garlic, sauté, stirring constantly, for 30 seconds.

Mix sugar and soy sauce together in small bowl till combined and add to pan.

Mix well to coat and stir-fry for three-4 mins.

Asparagus ought to be crisp-mild at this thing.

Serve.

35. Tofu Scramble

Serves four

What you'll need:

1 small onion, diced

2 tablespoons olive oil

1 lb enterprise enterprise tofu, crumbled (extra enterprise organization is incredible, too)

2 garlic cloves, minced

2 tablespoons dietary yeast flakes

1 tablespoon tamari

2 teaspoons Dijon mustard

1/2 teaspoon turmeric

1 teaspoon sage

1/four teaspoon basil

1/4 teaspoon salt

1/four teaspoon floor black pepper

1 medium tomatoes, chopped

What to do:

In a large saucepan on medium-immoderate warm temperature, sauté the onions in oil until translucent.

In a medium bowl, stir collectively the crumbled tofu, garlic, dietary yeast, tamari, mustard, turmeric, sage, basil, salt and pepper until nicely-combined.

Add tofu combination to onions and scramble till tofu is browned and all the liquid has evaporated.

Toss with tomatoes and serve right now.

36. Crispy Tofu Fingers

Serves 2

What you'll want:

12 ouncesextra enterprise tofu

4 oz.. Vegetarian oyster sauce or 4 ouncessweet and sour sauce or four ounces. Fish fry sauce (or different desired)

1 teaspoon vegetable oil

Salt

Garlic powder or one of a kind seasoning, as favored

What to do:

Coat a cookie sheet with oil.

Slice tofu lengthwise, about 1/4 inch thick, and pat dry.

Put the sauce proper into a dish, and dip each piece of tofu into the sauce, coating it well (I used barbecue sauce, and it changed into tasty).

Place the tofu at the cookie sheet in a unmarried layer (Pieces can be touching, however need to now not overlap).

Sprinkle on favored seasoning.

Bake at four hundred ranges F for 20 to 1/2-hour, counting on how crispy you want it.

Some human beings love it very chewy, on the identical time as others pick out it even as it is in spite of the fact that tender.

37. Mushroom Tofu Stroganoff

Serves 6

What you'll need:

four tablespoons butter

1 1/2 cups finely chopped onions

four garlic cloves, minced

1 teaspoon dill

2 teaspoons basil

1 1/2 lbs tofu, lessen into 1-inch cubes

2 teaspoons soy sauce

four cups sliced mushrooms

1/2 teaspoon salt

1/4 teaspoon cayenne

3 quarts water

1 lb dry fettuccine (attempt the spinach type)

1 cup sour cream (or easy yogurt)

1/2 cup finely chopped sparkling parsley

2 teaspoons poppy seeds

What to do:

Melt 2 tbls butter in huge frying pan. Sauté the onions, garlic, dill and basil.

After five minutes upload the tofu and preserve to prepare dinner dinner until tofu is well browned.

Add soy sauce and stir. Add mushrooms salt and cayenne.

Lower warmth and prepare dinner dinner some other five mins.

Add bitter cream and parsley to mushrooms. Mix well.

Melt ultimate 2 tbls butter in saucepan and add the poppy seeds.

Cook five-10 minutes. Pour onto noodles and toss.

38. Tofu Bites

Serves 6

What you'll want:

1 lb extrafirm decreased-fat water-packed tofu, tired and cut into half of-inch cubes

1 1/2 teaspoons vegetable oil

1 teaspoon darkish sesame oil

2 tablespoons low sodium soy sauce

1 tablespoon rice vinegar

What to do:

Place tofu on numerous layers of heavy-duty paper towels. Cover tofu with additional paper towels, and allow stand 5 mins, pressing occasionally.

Heat oils in a huge nonstick skillet over medium-excessive warmth. Add tofu; sauté 7 minutes or until browned.

Place in a bowl. Drizzle with soy sauce and vinegar; toss lightly to coat. Cover and sit back at the least 1 hour, stirring every now and then.

39. Rosemary-Lemon Baked Tofu

Serves four

What you'll need:

sixteen ouncesorganization tofu, pressed for half of-hour

1 teaspoon lemon zest, minced

1/4 cup clean lemon juice

2 tablespoons soy sauce

three tablespoons olive oil

1 tablespoon glowing rosemary, minced

1/4 teaspoon floor black pepper

What to do:

Preheat oven to 375 F.

Cut the tofu into 6 slices.

Use a baking dish as a way to preserve your tofu slices in a single single layer.

In the dish, wisk together the components for the marinade.

Add tofu slices and flip to coat on every sides.

Bake for 45-60 mins, turning as quickly as halfway vla cooking time. The longer it baked, the chewier it becomes.

Remove from oven and allow cool about 10 minutes.

Store leftovers in a box within the refrigerator for three-4 days.

40. Cheesy Tofu Strips

Serves 4

What you'll want:

1 1/2 cups spaghetti sauce, divided

1/3 cup dried breadcrumbs (simple or Italian fashion)

1/three cup finely grated parmesan cheese

14 ounces. Agency tofu (1 block) or 14 ounces extra employer tofu, worn-out (1 block)

1 cup shredded reduced-fats mozzarella cheese or 1 cup everyday mozzarella cheese

What to do:

Preheat oven to 325°F

Coat a nine-via-13-inch baking dish with cooking spray.

Spread half of cup of spaghetti sauce lightly round backside of dish.

On a plate, combine bread crumbs and parmesan cheese. Set apart.

Slice tofu in 1/2 of of lengthwise, then reduce every half of lengthwise into thirds.

Cut each piece lengthwise another time into halves to create 12 sticks.

Coat every stick in crumb/cheese mixture, and area in baking dish.

Cover the sticks with final spaghetti sauce and top with mozzarella. Bake 20 to 25 mins.

Tofu Breakfast Recipes

Mini Tofu Quiches

Although tofu is considered as being bland and having no actual taste, in reality is one of the maximum versatile food as it truly takes any flavor we want and that allows us to use all sorts of spices for flavor. These unique quiches are flavorful and truely scrumptious. Not to say that they have no crust so they're much less difficult to make.

Ingredients:

2 garlic cloves, minced

1 pink bell pepper, cored and diced

1 cup mushrooms, chopped

10 ozcompany tofu, worn-out and crumbled

1/4 cup soy milk

1 tablespoon cornstarch

1/8 teaspoon turmeric

1 leeks, chopped

three eggs

4 tablespoons butter

salt, pepper

Directions:

Grease your muffin tin barely with butter. Set apart.

Melt the last butter in a pan and stir within the leeks. Cook for five minutes, stirring often then upload the mushrooms and put together dinner a few different five minutes. Add a pinch of salt and pepper then the turmeric and cornstarch. Remove from heat and set apart to chill. Once chilled, stir inside the eggs, soy milk and tofu.

Spoon proper right into a greased muffin tin and bake inside the preheated oven at

350F for 30-40 minutes or till slightly golden brown.

Tofu and Apple Scramble

A super preference for breakfast, this scramble is flavorful and despite the fact that the aggregate may additionally furthermore have a weird sense, don't forget me after I say that apples flavor in reality as incredible in savory meals as they do in sweets.

Ingredients:

1 package deal company tofu, crumbled

2 tablespoons olive oil

half of of teaspoon onion powder

half of of teaspoon turmeric

1 teaspoon soy sauce

1 green apple, peeled and finely cubed

salt, pepper

Directions:

Heat the oil in a big heavy skillet and stir inside the crumbled tofu. Cook for 5 mins until the liquids begin to evaporate. Add the onion powder, turmeric, apple cubes and put together dinner dinner for 10 greater minutes, stirring all the times, until the apple is easy. Stay close to due to the reality the tofu has a tendency to stick to the lowest of the pan.

Stir in the soy sauce then dispose of from warmth. Add salt and freshly floor pepper if needed.

Serving recommendations:

Serve with a sprinkle of chopped corlander or parsley.

Spicy Tofu Frittata

Frittata makes an top notch desire for your morning food really as it gathers severa materials in a unmarried area, making it filling and attractive. This unique recipe yields a highly spiced version of frittata, however you may lower the warmth through decreasing the amount of spice.

Ingredients:

1 crimson onion, chopped

2 tablespoons coconut oil

1 package deal deal deal commercial enterprise enterprise tofu, cubed

2 garlic cloves, chopped

half of teaspoon turmeric

1/4 teaspoon cayenne pepper

1 purple bell pepper, cored and diced

1 green bell pepper, cored and diced

half of of cup diced tomatoes, worn-out

four eggs

salt, pepper

Directions:

Heat the olive oil in a big heavy skillet and sauté the onion for five mins until easy. Add the garlic and sauté 30 seconds until fragrant then stir within the tofu. Cook 5 mins until the beverages begin to evaporate then stir in the turmeric, cayenne pepper, bell peppers and tomatoes. Keep sautéing for 5-10 greater mins.

Beat the eggs with a pinch of salt and pepper in a bowl and pour the aggregate within the pan, over the tofu. Lower the warm temperature and cover the pan with a lid. Cook until the eggs coagulate and all of the veggies are cooked through, approximately 10-15 mins. If needed, flip the frittata as quickly as.

Serving hints:

Serve warmth together with your preferred sauce, together with tomato or garlic.

Tofu Scramble with Salsa

Juicy and highly spiced, this scramble is being the super choice for breakfast, specially whilst you're a vegetarian. All the spices used provide it a fragrant taste and the spiciness is being toned down by way of the use of the tomato salsa.

Ingredients:

2 tablespoons olive oil

1 small onion, finely chopped

1 package deal deal commercial enterprise employer tofu, crumbled

half teaspoon turmeric

1 teaspoon dietary yeast

1/eight teaspoon cayenne pepper

1/four teaspoon dried oregano

2 large tomatoes

1 garlic clove

half of teaspoon dried basil

salt, pepper

Directions:

Heat the olive oil in a large pan then stir within the cubed tofu and prepare dinner dinner till barely golden brown. Add the onion and hold cooking until mild. Stir within the turmeric, nutritional yeast, cayenne pepper and oregano. Add a pinch of salt if wanted and freshly ground pepper. Cook for five-10 mins till all the drinks have started out out to evaporate.

To make the salsa, peeled the tomatoes and reduce them into cubes. Drain the juices and blend the cubes with basil, garlic, salt and pepper.

Serving hints:

Serve the scrambled tofu crowned with tomato salsa.

Broccoli and Tofu Quiche

Quiches are basically savory brownies, however they have got the extraordinary advantage of being able to be made earlier of time then really reheated inside the morning for a fast breakfast. They also are very flexible and they'll be made with any of your favored vegetables.

Ingredients:

1 package deal pie crust dough

1 pound broccoli, trimmed and reduce into florets

2 green onions, chopped

1/2 teaspoon garlic powder

1 package deal deal commercial enterprise enterprise tofu, crumbled

half of of cup milk

1 pinch of nutmeg

4 eggs

1/4 cup grated Parmesan cheese

salt, pepper

Directions:

Grease a 9-inch round deep dish baking pan with a bit of butter and set apart.

Flour your strolling ground properly then roll out the dough. Transfer it into the pan and press it slightly along with your fingertips on the lowest and facets of the pan.

Spread the broccoli and tofu on the bottom of the pan.

Beat the eggs in a bowl with a pinch of salt, pepper and nutmeg. Add the garlic powder and inexperienced onions and pour the mixture over the veggies within the pan. Sprinkle grated Parmesan and bake inside the preheated oven at 350F for forty-50 minutes.

Serving hints:

Serve warmth or bloodless with an yogurt and garlic sauce.

Tofu Snack Recipes

Garlic Tofu Bites

Even if you could now not be a tofu fan, these bites will impress you. Tofu has the outstanding advantage of being infused with all kinds of spices and having a really remarkable texture. These particular bites are barely tangy, however a chunk highly spiced, caramelized and flavored with garlic.

Ingredients:

1/four cup low-sodium tamarind

6 garlic cloves, minced

juice from half of lime

1/2 of cup orange juice

1 teaspoon glowing grated ginger

2 tablespoons molasses

1 teaspoon curry powder

half of teaspoon garam masala

2 tablespoons cornstarch

1 pound organisation tofu, lessen into bite-duration pieces

1 cup sunflower seeds

salt, pepper

Directions:

In a saucepan, combo the tamarind paste, orange juice, garlic, lime juice, ginger, molasses, curry powder, garam masala, a pinch of salt and pepper. Bring to a boil then simmer on low warm temperature for five mins. Mix the cornstarch with 2 tablespoons water and stir it into the simmering combination. Cook 1 more minute till thickened. Let it cool to room temperature then combination inside the tofu quantities and marinade for two hours.

After hours, switch on your oven and set the temperature on immoderate. Take every piece of tofu and roll they all in sunflowers seeds. Arrange all of them on a baking tray coated with baking paper and bake inside the oven for 20-half of-hour or till caramelized and golden brown.

Serving recommendations:

Serve them clean, as they may be, chilled.

Tofu Chips

Tofu is virtually as flexible as potatoes. This recipe yields tofu chips and they will be scrumptious and flavorful due to all of the spices used. Of route, being so bendy, you may mess around with spices and use your chosen, it's far all as masses as you.

Ingredients:

1 pound organisation tofu

oil for frying

salt, pepper

Italian seasoning or some specific seasoning you need

Directions:

Finely slice the tofu. Season each slice with salt, freshly ground pepper and your preferred seasoning and allow them to sit down for 1/2 of-hour. Dry every slice with a paper towel.

Heat a small amount of oil in a heavy skillet and fry every slice of tofu on each factors till golden brown and crisp.

Serving guidelines:

Serve collectively with your chosen dip.

Tofu Kabobs

Being so bland in flavor, tofu can take quite lots the flavor of any spices used, this is the case with the ones kabobs. They are fragrant and delicious due to the usage of turmeric, chili and garlic, but they make and extremely good snack or why no longer, even a whole meal.

Ingredients:

1 pound organization tofu, reduce into small cubes

1/4 cup soy sauce

1 crimson chili pepper, chopped

4 garlic cloves, minced

2 tablespoons sesame oil

1 teaspoon rice vinegar

1 pinch of freshly ground pepper

Directions:

In a bowl, combine the soy sauce with pepper, garlic, sesame oil, vinegar and pepper. Mix well then stir inside the tofu cubes. Let them marinade for two hours then located the portions of tofu on skewers.

Heat a grill pan on medium flame and cook dinner dinner the tofu kabobs on all elements till barely golden brown and caramelized.

Serving guidelines:

Serve together together with your preferred dip.

Berry Tofu Smoothie

Yes, this is right! You can use tofu in drinks too, the very last texture being a whole lot richer and dense. Although it might now not have an impact on the taste hundreds, the use of tofu in this smoothie makes it healthier and affords it with enough nutrients to maintain you going till lunch.

Ingredients:

1 cup mixed berries

3 ozCorporation tofu, tired

1 banana, peeled

1 cup almond milk

Directions:

Combine all of the elements in a blender or meals processor and pulse till nicely mixed and easy.

Serving hints:

Add a teaspoon of flax seeds for added vitamins.

Tofu and Kale Bruschetta

Bruschetta is a high-quality possibility in your snacks because it is simple to make and you can use any additives you need. It is also healthy because the components are barely cooked so that they maintain their herbal flavors and nutrients.

Ingredients:

4 slices baguette

1 garlic clove, minced

2 tablespoons olive oil

1 kale leaf

3 ox tofu, crumbled

salt, pepper

Directions:

Heat a small pan over medium flame and upload 1 tablespoon olive oil. Stir inside the crumbled tofu and cook dinner dinner dinner till barely golden brown. Add the kale, chopped, and cook dinner dinner 1 extra minutes until actually easy. Season with a pinch of salt and pepper and set apart.

Mix the final oil with garlic and brush every slice of baguette. Toast the bread in a pan, on each side, till golden brown.

Spoon the tofu mixture over each slice.

Serving tips:

The tofu mixture bears even more spices, so be bold and use your favorite ones.

Tofu Salad Recipes

Tofu Avocado Salad

Avocado is one of the healthiest meals because it most effective carries healthy fat, which we need for our mind and to preserve our energy degree on a immoderate. It is likewise rich in proteins, so as a vegetarian, you need to include it into your weight loss program.

Ingredients:

1 bundle deal enterprise tofu, lessen into bite-period portions

1/2 of head lettuce, shredded

2 tablespoons sesame oil

half teaspoon turmeric

2 garlic cloves, minced

1 tablespoon rice vinegar

1/8 teaspoon chili flakes

1-2 avocados, peeled and reduce into slices

salt, pepper

juice from half of lemon

Directions:

Heat the sesame oil in a large frying pan and stir in the tofu. Cook till slightly golden brown then stir in the turmeric, garlic, chili flakes, vinegar. Cook 1 greater mins till fragrant then cast off from heat and permit it cool.

In a salad bowl, blend the lettuce with the avocado slices and lemon juice, similarly to salt and a pinch of pepper. Add the cooked tofu.

Serving recommendations:

Serve proper away, whilst nonetheless easy and fragrant. You can use arugula rather than lettuce.

Tofu Pasta Salad

Filling and healthful, this salad can be loved cold and it's miles fantastic for your lunch subject as it high-quality releases flavors in time.

Ingredients:

10 ozCorporation tofu, tired and cubed

2 tablespoons sesame oil

6 ouncesMacaroni noodles

1 small onion, sliced

1 red bell pepper, cored and sliced

2 garlic cloves, minced

4 ouncesmozzarella slices

2 tablespoons purple wine vinegar

2 tablespoons lemon juice

1 teaspoon soy sauce

half teaspoon oregano

2 tablespoons olive oil

salt, pepper

Directions:

Pour some cups of water in a pot, add a pinch of salt and convey to a boil. Throw within the macaroni noodles and prepare dinner until simply al dente.

Heat the sesame oil in a huge frying pan and stir inside the tofu. Cook, stirring frequently, until golden brown on all factors. Remove the tofu from the pan and in the same oil, sauté the onion for three-4 minutes, then add the garlic and red bell pepper and cook dinner 2 extra minutes. Put the tofu once more into the pan, then add the noodles. Set apart to loosen up.

In a small bowl, whisk the vinegar with the lemon juice, oregano, olive oil, a pinch of salt and pepper.

Drizzle the dressing over the salad and blend well.

Serving suggestions:

It is remarkable served 1 few hours later, after all the flavors have infused together.

Tofu Spinach Salad

Spinach and tofu come collectively in this recipe to create a scrumptious, sparkling salad, with strong flavors and packed with nutrients and vitamins.

Ingredients:

half of of cup commercial enterprise business enterprise tofu, lessen into small cubes

2 cups little one spinach leaves

1 purple bell pepper, cored and sliced

1 carrot, grated

1 garlic clove

1/8 teaspoon chili flakes

2 tablespoons lemon juice

2 tablespoons olive oil

salt, pepper

Directions:

Mix the spinach with tofu, carrot and bell pepper in a bowl, then upload the garlic, lemon juice, chili flakes, oil and season with a pinch of salt and pepper.

Serving guidelines:

Serve proper away to ensure you enjoy all the flavors

Tofu and Quinoa Salad

Since tofu has this form of slight taste, it could be mixed with a few issue without the worry of carrying out with a few component that may not taste proper. This salad is healthy and full of fibers and vitamins and has the gain of being even better after some hours so that you could make it in the morning and feature it organized for a fast lunch.

Ingredients:

1 cup cooked quinoa

6 ozCorporation tofu, lessen into small cubes

1 ripe avocado, peeled and sliced

five ozcherry tomatoes, halved

half of cup canned sweet corn, tired

1 shallot, finely sliced

2 tablespoons lemon juice

2 tablespoons olive oil

salt, pepper

Directions:

In a bowl, combination together the quinoa, tofu, avocado, tomatoes, corn and shallot. Gently stir inside the lemon juice, olive oil and a pinch of salt and freshly ground pepper.

Serving tips:

For extra freshness, upload a handful of chopped coriander leaves.

Soba Noodles and Tofu Salad

Noodles are very Asian and so are the flavors used in this salad. It is wholesome and peppery, however exciting and perfect for summer time day at the same time as you certainly want a few issue mild.

Ingredients:

eight ouncessoba noodles

4 ozinexperienced peas

1 carrot, peeled and reduce into wonderful sticks

2 tablespoons rice vinegar

1 teaspoon miso paste

2 tablespoons olive oil

1 tablespoon soy sauce

1 teaspoon glowing grated ginger

1 teaspoon honey

five ozcompany tofu, reduce into cubes

1 cup infant spinach leaves

1/four teaspoon purple pepper flakes

salt, pepper

Directions:

Pour some cups of water in a huge pot, upload a pinch of salt and produce to a boil. Cook till without a doubt al dente then, in the ultimate minute of cooking, throw inside the peas and carrot as well. Drain and set apart to kick back.

In a small bowl, combination the vinegar, soy sauce, miso paste, ginger and honey. Set apart.

Heat the olive oil in a large frying pan and stir within the tofu cubes. Cook, stirring regularly, until golden brown on all facets. Add the spinach and purple pepper flakes and put together dinner 1 greater minute. Remove from warmth and placed the in a bowl to loosen up.

Stir in the soba noodles, together with the peas, carrot and the dressing you whisked in advance. Mix lightly to evenly coat.

Serving suggestions:

Serve with a sprinkle of sunflower or pumpkin seeds for extra texture.

Tofu Soup Recipes

Hot and Sour Tofu Soup

There isn't always whatever better than a bowl of heat soup to make you revel in higher in case you are ill. This precise recipe yields a exceedingly spiced, but bitter soup so that you can wake up your flavor buds and senses.

Ingredients:

1 tablespoon curry paste

1 stick lemongrass

four cups vegetable inventory

1 red chili, crushed

2 potatoes, peeled and cubed

1 shallot, chopped

five ozbutton mushrooms

1 package deal business enterprise tofu, reduce into cubes

1 cup cherry tomatoes, halved

salt, pepper

juice from 1 lime

Directions:

Pour the inventory in a large soup pot and bring to a boil. Add the curry paste, lemongrass, purple chili, potatoes and prepare dinner for 5 minutes. Throw inside the final factors and cook dinner dinner any other 10 mins. Just earlier than removing from warmness, blend inside the lime juice.

Serving pointers:

Serve while nevertheless heat, sprinkled with chopped coriander.

Tofu and Mushroom Soup

A snug soup that allows you to awaken your taste buds. It is simple to make, however its texture is silky and the flavor is divine.

Ingredients:

5 cups vegetable inventory

1 package deal deal business enterprise tofu, cubed

1 cup sliced mushrooms

2 cups toddler spinach leaves

2 green onions, sliced

1 tablespoon sesame oil

salt, pepper

Directions:

Pour the stock in a huge pot and bring to a boil. Stir in the tofu, mushrooms, a pinch of salt and pepper. Cook for 5 minutes then upload the spinach and onions. Cook some unique 5 minutes. Before disposing of from warm temperature, drizzle the sesame oil.

Serving tips:

Serve with a beneficiant sprinkle of chopped coriander.

Thai Vegetable and Tofu Soup

The greater veggies, the merrier. This soup has the gain of now not cooking the veggies an excessive amount of, so all the nutrients and nutrients are preserved.

Ingredients:

1 cup oyster mushrooms, sliced

1 inch galangal, peeled

1/2 of of inch ginger, peeled

1 onion, sliced

1 lemongrass stalk

1 red pepper, overwhelmed

1 huge carrot, reduce into outstanding sticks

eight ouncescompany tofu, lessen into small cubes

2 tablespoons coconut oil

2 lime leaves

4 cups water

1 teaspoon soy sauce

salt, pepper

2 tablespoons chopped Thai basil leaves

Directions:

Grate the galangal and ginger and mix it with the mushrooms, carrot, onion, lemongrass, lime leaves and crimson pepper in a pot. Cover with water, upload a pinch of salt and bring to a boil. Simmer on low warmth for 10 minutes.

Heat the coconut oil in a large frying pan and sauté the tofu cubes for 10-15 minutes, mixing all of the time, till golden brown and crisp. Transfer the tofu into the ultra-modern soup and put together dinner five more mins. Add the soy sauce and basil then simmer 1 extra minute. Remove the pink pepper, lime leaves and lemongrass earlier than serving.

Serving tips:

Serve warmth, sprinkled with masses of coriander leaves, chopped, or greater basil.

Spinach and Tofu Soup

We all recognise how healthy spinach is, but for a few reason we maintain keeping off it, the primary motive being that we do not recognise a way to prepare dinner dinner dinner it so it tastes correct. This soup, however, gives us a delicious alternative. It is wealthy, a piece relatively spiced, however not too much and it is filling, ideal for those cold days even as you need some warmth.

Ingredients:

2 tablespoons vegetable oil

1 onion, chopped

2 garlic cloves, minced

three cups water

3 cups vegetable inventory

2 tomatoes, peeled and chopped

4 green onions, finely sliced

four cups spinach leaves, coarsely chopped

10 ozcorporation tofu, reduce into small cubes

2 teaspoons soy sauce

salt, pepper

Directions:

Heat the oil in a big soup pot and stir in the onion. Sauté for 5 minutes then add the garlic and put together dinner 1 more minute. Pour inside the water and vegetable stock and convey to a boil. Stir in the chopped tomatoes and tofu. Cover with a lid and simmer for 10 mins.

Mix in the green onion, spinach, a touch of salt and pepper. Cook 10 greater minutes.

Remove from warmth and mix inside the soy sauce.

Serving tips:

Serve heat sprinkled with chopped coriander or parsley and some Parmesan shavings.

Carrot and Tofu Soup

Although slightly candy because of the carrot, this soup is first rate and its deliciousness lies in its simplicity.

Ingredients:

2 cups vegetable shares

1 pound carrots, peeled and sliced

1 small onion, chopped

2 garlic cloves, minced

1 teaspoon easy grated ginger

1 teaspoon Thai curry paste

four oz.Organization tofu, cubed

salt, pepper

Directions:

Put the carrots, inventory, onion, garlic and ginger in a small soup pot and convey to a boil. Simmer on low to medium warmness for 20 mins then stir in the tofu and cook 10 greater mins. Stir in the curry paste, a pinch of salt and freshly ground pepper then, using an immersion blender, puree the combination until easy and creamy.

Serving hints:

Serve warm, sprinkled with chopped parsley and some mint leaves.

Tofu Main Dish Recipes

Tofu Burger

Being a vegetarian nowadays does no longer mean you cannot however revel in all the styles of food in reality absolutely everyone else does. This recipe yields such moist and delicious burgers that even a meat eater will revel in them.

Ingredients:

2 kilos company tofu

2 teaspoons soy sauce

1 teaspoon oregano

four garlic cloves, minced

1 teaspoon dried basil

1/2 of of teaspoon onion powder

2 tablespoons red miso paste

salt, pepper

Directions:

Cut the tofu into skinny slices. Put the slices in a bowl. Sprinkle the final materials and gently toss to softly coat the tofu slices. Cover with plastic wrap and positioned inside the refrigerator to marinade for 2 hours.

Heat a grill pan over medium flame. Grill each tofu slice on every aspects till golden brown and aromatic.

Serving guidelines:

Serve among burger rolls collectively collectively with your preferred toppings.

Vegetable Tofu Stir-Fry

Stir-fries are short to make and delicious, due to the fact the greens aren't cooked prolonged enough to lose their nutrients and nutrients, so that you can ensure your meal is filling and it has sufficient nutrients to hold you going until the following meal.

Ingredients:

2 cups cooked white rice

2 tablespoons soy sauce

2 tablespoons hoisin sauce

1 tablespoon balsamic vinegar

2 tablespoons cornstarch

2 tablespoons sesame oil

four inexperienced onions, sliced

three garlic cloves, chopped

1 teaspoon grated ginger

1 cup shiitake mushrooms, chopped

2/3 cup snow peas

1 package deal business enterprise tofu, reduce into small cubes

salt, pepper to taste

Directions:

In a small bowl, combo the two sauces, balsamic vinegar, cornstarch and half cup of water then set apart until use.

Heat the sesame oil in a wok over medium to excessive flame and stir in the inexperienced onions, garlic and ginger. Mix properly and sauté 30 seconds. Throw in the mushrooms and put together dinner three mins then upload the snow peas and prepare dinner 2 more mins. Pour in the sauce you whisked earlier and blend well until thick. Stir within the cubed tofu and prepare dinner dinner 2 more mins.

Serving recommendations:

Serve sprinkled with green onions.

Grilled Tofu with Mixed Vegetables

Grilling tofu is first rate thinking about you could marinade it earlier than so it tastes heavenly with its natural sweetness and smoky grilled taste.

Ingredients:

1 package deal greater-organization tofu

1 big eggplant, finely sliced lengthwise

2 zucchinis, finely sliced lengthwise

1 purple onion, coarsely sliced

1 purple bell pepper

1 cup cherry tomatoes

2 tablespoons olive oil

1 teaspoon dried oregano

1 teaspoon dried basil

1 tablespoon balsamic vinegar

salt, pepper

Directions:

Cut the tofu into thin slices. Season with freshly ground pepper and grill on a heated grill pan until golden brown on every aspects.

Season the greens with salt and pepper as nicely then brush all of them with olive oil. Cook them at the grill as well then switch proper right into a bowl and upload the balsamic vinegar, oregano and basil.

Serve the tofu garnished with greens.

Serving tips:

You can make them in advance and allow them to marinade for two-3 hours as that could decorate the flavors.

Thai Tofu Curry

Saucy and flavorful, this curry is fantastic for lunch or dinner. It is likewise easy to make and delicious, perfect to experience with a slice of smooth bread, dipping into the sauce.

Ingredients:

2 cups cubed pumpkin

half of of cup coconut milk

2 teaspoons curry paste

1 small onion, chopped

1 cup mushrooms, sliced

half cup inexperienced peas

10 ozCompany tofu, cut into cubes

2 tablespoons vegetable oil

salt, pepper

Directions:

Pour the coconut milk in a saucepan and stir within the curry paste. Add the pumpkin and onion and bring to a boil, then simmer on low warmth for 5-10 minutes. Mix inside the chopped mushrooms and maintain cooking 5 extra minutes. Add the peas and cook dinner dinner till all the vegetables are gentle and easy.

Heat the vegetable oil in a frying pan and stir in the cubed tofu. Cook for a couple of minutes till golden brown on all sides. Add the tofu into the curry, season with salt and pepper and remove from warmth.

Serving pointers:

Serve with cooked jasmine rice and naan bread.

Tofu Parmigiana

A conventional Italian dish, Parmigiana moreover may be made with tofu and also you could no longer even be conscious the difference from the conventional eggplant one.

Ingredients:

1/2 of cup breadcrumbs

half of of cup grated Parmesan cheese

1 teaspoon dried oregano

1 teaspoon dried basil

1 package deal agency tofu

2 tablespoons more virgin olive oil

1 cup tomato sauce

2 garlic cloves

1 cup shredded mozzarella

salt, pepper

Directions:

In a bowl, combine the breadcrumbs with 1/2 of of of the Parmesan, oregano, basil, salt and pepper.

Slice the tofu into 1/4 inch thick quantities then coat each slice with breadcrumbs mixture.

Heat the olive oil in a frying pan and prepare dinner the tofu slices on every elements until golden brown.

In each other bowl or big cup, mix the tomato sauce with garlic, a pinch of salt and pepper.

Take a small deep dish baking pan and start layering the tofu with tomato sauce within the pan. End with a tomato layer then top with the closing Parmesan and shredded mozzarella. Bake within the preheated oven at 400F for 20-half-hour.

Serving pointers:

Serve slightly heat, sprinkled with chopped parsley.

Tofu Wraps

Easy to make and healthful, the ones wraps are scrumptious and percent best nutrients and fibers, being able to give you an electricity improve at the equal time as you need it.

Ingredients:

1 package deal deal agency tofu

2 tablespoons soy sauce

1 tablespoon lemon juice

1/four teaspoon garlic powder

1/eight teaspoon cayenne pepper

1 red bell pepper, cored and sliced

four green onion, coarsely chopped

1/2 of of cup chopped coriander

8 tortilla flour

eight lettuce leaves

salt, pepper

Directions:

Cut the tofu into small cubes. Transfer into a bowl and blend within the lemon juice, garlic powder, cayenne pepper, soy sauce and ground black pepper. Mix nicely to frivolously coat the cubes. Add the final factors and spoon the aggregate on tortillas. Top with a lettuce leaf and wrap tight.

Serving recommendations:

Serve with peanut butter if you want it.

Tofu Filets

Simple, but scrumptious, the ones filets are the show that simplicity is higher every so often.

Ingredients:

1 package organization tofu, sliced

1 tablespoon soy sauce

1 tablespoon tamari sauce

1 teaspoon Cajun seasoning

Directions:

Put the tofu slices in a bowl and blend inside the soy sauce, tamari sauce and seasoning. Let it marinade for two-3 hours then put together dinner at the grill pan every slice, on each aspects until golden brown.

Serving recommendations:

You can use any seasoning you want to create your very own dish. Serve them amongst bread slices, topped with tomato slices and lettuce leaves.

Sweet Potato and Tofu Stew

Stews are superb in some unspecified time in the future of wintry weather. Cooked on low heat, they release super flavors and the sauce is thick and flavorful, ideal to comfort you on a cold wintry climate day.

Ingredients:

1 cup pumpkin cubes

10 ozorganization tofu, cubed

1 celery stalk, chopped

1 small zucchini, diced

2 red onions, chopped

1 cup mushrooms, sliced

1 carrot, sliced

2 sweet potatoes, peeled and cubed

2-three cups vegetable stock

1 teaspoon smooth grated ginger

salt, pepper

Directions:

Put the tofu, celery, onions, mushrooms, carrot, ginger and stock in a pot and convey to a boil. Add a pinch of salt if wished and freshly floor pepper and simmer on low heat for 1/2 of-hour. Stir inside the pumpkin and candy potatoes and put together dinner dinner 15 more minutes on low warmth.

Serving recommendations:

Serve warmth with a dollop of sparkling cooking cream and a sprinkle of parsley.

Tofu Lasagna

A remake of the conventional lasagna, this particular one taste in truth as actual, while now not having any kind of meat. It may be a chunk more time eating to make, but it is well in reality definitely worth the time sometimes.

Ingredients:

eight lasagna noodles

2 tablespoons olive oil

1 onion, chopped

1 cup mushrooms, sliced

2 garlic cloves, minced

1 package frozen spinach, defrosted and squeezed to get rid of the liquid

2 cups tomato sauce

10 ouncesorganization tofu, crumbled

1 teaspoon dried oregano

1 teaspoon dried basil

2 cups mozzarella cheese

salt, pepper

Directions:

Cook the lasagna noodles as said on the package deal.

Heat the olive oil in a heavy skillet and stir in the onion. Sauté five minutes then add the mushrooms and put together dinner till the liquids begins offevolved to evaporate. Add the minced garlic and spinach and hold sautéing for five-10 mins. Stir within the tomato sauce, oregano and basil then season with salt and pepper. Remove from warmth and set aside.

To finish the lasagna, take a deep dish baking pan and layer the lasagna noodles with the sauce you made in advance and crumbled tofu. Finish with a tomato layer and pinnacle with mozzarella cheese.

Bake within the preheated oven at 375F for forty five minutes or till the cheese has melted and appears effervescent and golden brown.

Serving tips:

Serve it slightly heat with a dollop of sour cream in case you choice.

Spaghetti and Tofu Meatballs

Italians and their pasta are inseparable. But I have to admit that this dish is honestly scrumptious in order that they've to be expertise a few aspect. These meatballs, made with tofu in preference to meat are wet and quite delicious.

Ingredients:

1 package deal business enterprise tofu

1 cup breadcrumbs

2 tablespoons tahini paste

1 tablespoon soy sauce

1 tablespoon Dijon mustard

half of teaspoon garlic powder

2 tablespoons vegetable oil

four cups tomato sauce

1 teaspoon oregano

1 teaspoon basil

10 ouncesspaghetti

half cup grated Parmesan

salt, pepper

Directions:

Put the tofu in a food processor and pulse until crumbled. Add the breadcrumbs, tahini paste, Dijon, soy sauce and garlic powder, in addition to the oil. Pulse till nicely blended and it comes collectively as a dough. Season with salt and pepper if favored then form into small balls.

Heat a small amount of vegetable oil in a huge frying pan and prepare dinner dinner the balls on every detail for 2 minutes or until golden brown.

To make the sauce, pour the tomato sauce in a saucepan. Bring to a boil, then stir in the oregano, basil and tofu balls. Cook on low warmth for 10 mins.

Pour some cups of water in a huge pot, add a pinch of salt and convey to a boil. Throw inside the spaghetti and cook dinner until absolutely al dente.

Serve the spaghetti topped with tomato sauce and tofu balls.

Serving Suggestions:

Top with chopped parsley really before serving.

Tofu Chili

Spicy and saucy, this dish is fantastic for lunch, but furthermore for dinner. It is filling, quite smooth to make and the flavors are in particular balanced.

Ingredients:

1 package deal deal extra-commercial enterprise employer tofu, reduce into cubes

1 purple bell pepper, cored and sliced

1 green bell pepper, cored and sliced

1 inexperienced chili, deseeded and chopped

2 tablespoons sesame oil

1 teaspoon coriander powder

half of teaspoon cumin powder

1 onion, chopped

1 teaspoon garlic powder

1 teaspoon grated ginger

1 tablespoon soy sauce

salt, pepper

Directions:

Heat the sesame oil in a heavy pan and stir in the tofu. Cook till golden brown on all aspects. Add the cumin powder, ginger, garlic, coriander powder and onion. Sauté on low heat until the onion is mild then upload the chili and bell peppers. Cook till the peppers are slightly smooth then stir in the soy sauce and a pinch of freshly ground pepper.

Serving tips:

Serve warmness sprinkled with chopped coriander and a dollop of glowing cream or yogurt.

Italian Baked Tofu

Having those strong Italian flavors, this dish is not for all of us, however in case you revel in smooth taste and this Italian sense, then it is the recipe for you.

Ingredients:

three garlic cloves

3 tablespoons olive oil

2 tablespoons balsamic vinegar

2 tablespoons white wine

1 teaspoon dried basil

1 teaspoon dried oregano

1 teaspoon dried marjoram

1 bundle deal deal corporation tofu, sliced

freshly floor pepper

Directions:

In a bowl, blend the garlic, with vinegar, basil, marjoram, oregano and white wine. Toss within the tofu slices, being cautious to coat all of them then marinade for 1 hour.

Arrange each slice on a baking tray coated with parchment paper then crush they all with olive oil. Bake within the preheated oven at 400F for 20 minutes on one aspect. Flip them over and prepare dinner dinner dinner every different 10 mins.

Serving guidelines:

Serve them with a glowing salad on one facet or use them to make sandwiches.

Tofu Tandoori

Spicy and complete of robust flavors, this tandoori isn't always for the faint of coronary coronary heart. However, in case you need this form of meals, it is absolutely nicely in reality really worth a try to make your non-public at home as you may manipulate the quantity of spices.

Ingredients:

2 tablespoons coconut oil

1 teaspoon coriander powder

1 teaspoon cumin powder

1 teaspoon turmeric

half teaspoon cayenne pepper

1 teaspoon grated ginger

1 teaspoon garam masala

1 cup Greek style yogurt

1 tablespoons lemon juice

2 garlic cloves, minced

1 package company tofu, cubed

salt, pepper

Directions:

Mix all of the spices, yogurt, lemon juice and garlic, further to salt and pepper in a bowl then combination in the cubes of tofu. Let them marinade for two hours then skewer then on timber skewer and grill them in a warmth grill pan, brushed with oil. Cook on all elements until golden brown.

Serving guidelines:

Serve with lime slices and a easy salad on one aspect.

Tofu Manicotti

Italians are masters at making pasta so this recipe is a masterpiece as it's miles filling, it has enough vegetables and sufficient spice, it's miles saucy and juicy, certainly delicious for any meal of the day.

Ingredients:

2 tablespoons olive oil

1 teaspoon dried basil

half of of teaspoon dried oregano

half of teaspoon garlic powder

15 ouncesCorporation tofu, crumbled

1 package frozen spinach, thawed and squeezed to dispose of the liquids.

1 field manicotti shells

2 cups tomato sauce

1 cup mozzarella, shredded

salt, pepper

Directions:

Cook the manicotti shells consistent with the instructions at the field.

Put the tofu in a meals processor and pulse till well combined and crumbled.

Add the rest of the substances, besides the tomato sauce and mozzarella. Season the filling with salt and pepper then fill every shells with sufficient tofu combination. Arrange the manicotti in a deep dish baking pan, then cover with tomato sauce and top with mozzarella.

Bake inside the preheated oven at 375F for 30-40 minutes.

Serving hints:

Serve warm, on the identical time because the cheese remains gooey, with a dollop of cream if you want.

Tofu Coconut Curry

Flavorful and creamy, this curry is exquisite to be served with naan bread and sticky rice, garnished with a lime wedge.

Ingredients:

4 tablespoons olive oil

1 package greater-corporation tofu, reduce into small cubes

1 tablespoon sparkling grated ginger

3 garlic cloves, minced

1 teaspoon curry powder

1 small onion, chopped

2 huge carrot, sliced

2 cups canned diced tomatoes

1 cup vegetable inventory

1 cup coconut milk

2 cups cooked basmati rice

salt, pepper

Directions:

Heat the olive oil in a heavy skillet and sauté the onion until smooth and translucent. Add the tofu and put together dinner dinner till golden brown, then stir in the ginger, carrots, tomatoes, coconut milk and vegetable stock. Bring to a boil then simmer on low warmth for 20 mins or until the liquid begins offevolved to evaporate and the sauce is creamy and wealthy. Season with salt and pepper and take away from warmth.

Serving pointers:

Serve on basmati rice, garnished with a lime wedge and sprinkled with hundreds of chopped coriander.

Tofu Sloppy Joes

Rich and moist, this dish is great for sandwiches, layered among burger buns with cheese and your chosen toppings. The appropriate statistics is that you may be a vegetarian and though experience it because it best has tofu, however the distinction is narrow because of which includes spices to make it flavor heavenly.

Ingredients:

2 tablespoons olive oil

four garlic cloves, minced

1 bundle more-employer tofu, crumbled

1 teaspoon dried oregano

1/2 teaspoon dried basil

1 onion, chopped

2 cups pasta sauce

1 teaspoon Dijon mustard

1 teaspoon brown sugar

salt, pepper

Directions:

Heat the olive oil in a large heavy saucepan and stir within the onion. Sauté for 5 minutes till mild and translucent then upload the tofu, garlic, oregano and basil. Cook on low heat for 2 minutes without a doubt to release flavors then blend in the pasta sauce, mustard and brown sugar. Bring to a boil and simmer on low warmness until thick, about 20-half-hour.

Season with salt and pepper and cast off from warm temperature.

Serving suggestions:

Serve in burger buns, topped with a slice of cheese.

Cilantro and Lime Grilled Tofu

Grilling tofu is the very first-class way of cooking it, but additionally one of the tastiest because of the fact the tofu is being marinated first then cooked on the grill.

Ingredients:

1 package organization-tofu, tired and decrease into slices

juice from1 lime

2 tablespoons olive oil

1 teaspoon garlic powder

1/2 teaspoon chili powder

2 tablespoons glowing chopped cilantro

half of of of teaspoon cumin seeds

1 pinch of nutmeg

salt, pepper if wanted

Directions:

In a bowl, combination the olive oil with the garlic powder, chili, cilantro, lime juice, cumin seeds and nutmeg. Toss within the tofu slices and mix them spherical to lightly coat every slice. Let them marinade for 2 hours.

Heat a grill pan over medium flame then cook dinner dinner dinner each slice of tofu on the grill, on every factors, till golden brown.

Serving suggestions:

Serve them with a sparkling salad on one side or your favored dip.

Sweet and Sour Tofu

Reading the materials, you'll be surprised by means of the use of the amount of honey used, but do now not be do away with with the beneficial resource of that. The very last end result isn't always that candy, but the honey makes it more flavorful and it permits beautify the opposite flavors.

Ingredients:

1 bundle company tofu, sliced

2 tablespoons olive oil

juice from 1 massive lemon

1/four cup honey

1/four cup soy sauce

1 teaspoon grated ginger

three garlic cloves, minced

Directions:

In a bowl, mixture the olive oil with the lemon juice, honey, soy sauce, ginger and garlic. Toss in the tofu slices and lightly coat them with sauce. Let them marinade for two hours.

Heat a grill pan over medium flame. Take each slice of tofu and scrape down the marinade if it is too much. Cook the tofu on the grill, on each side, till golden brown, about four-5 minutes, relying to your grill.

Serving pointers:

Serve warm, with a glowing salad on one aspect or use to make sandwiches along side your favored toppings.

Saag Tofu

Saag is exquisite to be served with naan bread or rice and this model is so creamy and saucy that each one you want to do is dip a slice of bread in it and revel in its lovable flavors awakening your flavor buds.

Ingredients:

1 bundle deal corporation tofu, tired

2 tablespoons vegetable oil

1 onion, chopped

2 garlic cloves, minced

1 teaspoon grated ginger

1 teaspoon curry powder

half of of teaspoon ground cumin

1 pound spinach leaves

1 cup easy yogurt

salt, pepper

Directions:

Heat the oil in a heavy saucepan and stir within the tofu. Cook for 5-10 mins until slightly golden brown. Stir in the onion and garlic and cook dinner 5 more mins, stirring regularly so it doesn't stick with the lowest of the pan. Add the ginger and the spinach, chopped and prepare dinner dinner for 6 more minutes.

Mix the yogurt with curry powder and cumin then pour it into the saucepan. Season with salt and freshly floor pepper if you preference and bring to a boil once more. Simmer 2 greater minutes then do away with from warmth.

Serving tips:

Serve over jasmine rice and eat with naan bread.

Tofu Veggie Loaf

Loaf is a outstanding possibility for lunch bins as it may be made way ahead and frozen then reheated even as you need a slice or packed on your lunch container. This model no longer first-rate makes use of tofu, but furthermore plenty of veggies and spices so it is scrumptious and flavorful.

Ingredients:

2 tablespoons olive oil

1 onion, chopped

2 carrots, peeled and grated

1/4 cup chopped parsley

2 packages employer tofu

1 cup bread crumbs

2 eggs

1/2 cup tomato sauce

1 teaspoon soy sauce

1 teaspoon Worcestershire sauce

half of of teaspoon garlic powder

half of of of teaspoon dried oregano

salt, pepper

Directions:

Line a nine-inch loaf pan with baking paper and set aside.

Preheat your oven at 350F.

Heat the oil in a huge frying pan and stir in the chopped onion, carrots, garlic powder and chopped parsley and prepare dinner dinner 10 minutes till gentle. Remove from warmth.

Drain the tofu properly and placed it right into a food processor. Pulse till well crumbled. Mix within the onion mixture from earlier, bread crumbs, eggs, tomato sauce, soy sauce and Worcestershire sauce, as well as dried oregano, salt and a pinch of pepper. Mix properly then spoon this batter into your protected loaf pan.

Cook in the oven for 1 hour. Let it quiet down definitely earlier than getting rid of from the pan and lowering.

Serving tips:

It is outstanding served on mashed potatoes or with simplest a easy salad on one facet.

Tofu Dessert Recipes

Tofu Chocolate Cheesecake

Cheesecake is a traditional, but if you are vegan, it's miles surely not part of your plans for dessert. Unless you are making this model that uses tofu in area of cream cheese. It is virtually as creamy and scrumptious, with an extreme chocolate taste, however also a sensitive creaminess.

Ingredients:

Crust:

1 1/2 of cups graham crackers

2 tablespoons powdered sugar

four tablespoons vegan buttery unfold, melted

Filling:

1 2/three cups sugar

1/3 cup soy milk

10 ouncesdark chocolate, chopped

2 packages silken tofu, nicely drained

4 tablespoons cocoa powder

15 ozsoy cream cheese

2 teaspoons vanilla extract

1 pinch of salt

Directions:

To make the crust: Put the cracker sin a food processor and pulse until well crumbled. Add the sugar and melted butter and pulse until it comes together. Line a 9-inch round cake pan with baking paper then spread the crust on the lowest of the pan and press it with your fingertips well. Set aside.

To make the filling: Put the tofu in a meals processor together with the sugar, milk, cocoa powder, cream cheese and vanilla. Pulse until well combined then stir in the melted chocolate.

Spoon the combination into the pan over the crust.

Bake inside the preheated oven at 350F for 1 hour.

Serving pointers:

Serve cold with a dollop of clean cream or whipped cream.

Pumpkin Tofu Cheesecake

Spiced, creamy and fragrant, this cheesecake redefines the notion of perfectly baked. It's no longer a long way from the traditional version of pumpkin cheesecake, however the tofu offers it more texture and the flavors come collectively in a nicely balanced way.

Ingredients:

Crust:

1 half of of cups graham crackers

6 tablespoons butter

Filling:

2 kilos silken tofu

1 cup canned pumpkin puree

1 cup sugar

2 eggs

1 teaspoon cinnamon

1/2 of teaspoon floor ginger

1/2 teaspoon floor cloves

10 ozCream cheese

2 teaspoons vanilla extract

Directions:

To make the crust: Put the crackers in a food processor and pulse until properly crumbled, then mix within the melted butter. Transfer the aggregate proper into a 9-inch spherical pan and press it down on the lowest and factors of the pan together along with your fingertips. Set aside.

To make the filling: Put the tofu in a food processor with the cream cheese and pulse until easy and nicely mixed. Add the sugar, pumpkin puree, eggs, spices and vanilla.

Pour the mixture into the pan over the crust and bake in the preheated oven at 350F for 1 hour.

Serving recommendations:

Serve chilled, crowned with whipped cream and sprinkled with cinnamon powder.

Tofu Chocolate Mousse

Chocolate mousse is surely some aspect we all crave for. Airy, creamy and wealthy, the chocolate mousse is a delight for our flavor buds. This unique model has plenty extra texture because of the tofu, but it tastes definitely as particular.

Ingredients:

1 cup dark chocolate, chopped

10 ozsilken tofu, tired

half cup soy milk

1 teaspoon vanilla extract

Directions:

Melt the chocolate in the microwave a few seconds.

Put the tofu in a food processor, then upload the melted chocolate, milk and vanilla. Pulse till clean and creamy then pass the combination through a exceptional sieve for a higher texture, but it is truely not a necessary step if you do no longer thoughts the grainy texture.

Spoon into serving bowls or glasses and refrigerate for some hours in advance than serving.

Serving suggestions:

Serve chilled and well set, with a dollop of glowing whipped cream. It additionally can be served with any shape of fruit gelee.

Tofu Peanut Butter Pie

Peanut butter pie is delicious and creamy, however adding tofu it will become a miles extra healthy version, without changing the taste masses, however being vegan and full of vitamins and fibers.

Ingredients:

10 ouncesSilken tofu

2/three cup peanut butter

half cup sugar

2 tablespoons soy milk

1 teaspoon vanilla extract

1 pie crust, baked

Directions:

Put the tofu in a food processor. Add the peanut butter, sugar, soy milk and vanilla and method until the mixture is simple and creamy. Spoon the aggregate into your baked pie crust and refrigerate a few hours before serving.

www.ingramcontent.com/pod-product-compliance
Lightning Source LLC
Chambersburg PA
CBHW060225030426
42335CB00014B/1340